ALOE VERA.

EVERY THING YOU

NEED TO KNOW.

PLANTING

PRESERVATION

HEALTH BENEFITS

The Aloevera Plant; An Overview

Aloe vera plants such as Aloe vera barbadensis are known for their medicinal use, various kinds of ailments and ointments are available for burns, rashes and cuts. They are use in various beauty preparations to give your skin a beautiful look. Aloe Vera plants are now found in various countries and have been commonly accepted as folk medicines. This plant can also be grown as an indoor plant but may need re-potting as it grows very large. Aloe Vera Plant is also known as medicinal aloe, medicine plant or burn plant. The name comes from the Arabic "Alloeh", meaning bitter because of the bitter yellow liquid that is found between the gel and the leaf skin. Aloe Vera plant looks like cactus, but is actually a member of the lily family. It grows in warm places like Asia, Africa and some parts of America and Europe that are warm. Aloe vera plants are prized for the gel substance inside their leaves which is used for many types of medicinal purposes (medicinal aloe vera).

Growing aloe vera plants can be something anyone can do and it lets a person keep an aloe plant on hand for whenever they need a little aloe vera gel. Aloe Vera plants are very easy to care for. They withstand quite a bit in my opinions. They do need a lot of sunlight, so it is best to keep them in a window that gets lots of sun, unless you are in an especially cold climate. They do need to be kept warm and get plenty of light, because they can die from exposure to cold. The plant is beneficial for uterus, liver, ulcers, colon and hemorrhoids disorders. Aloe vera not only provides healing effect to the person but it also returns the bowls to the normal position. They are easy to grow indoors and outdoors. However, growing aloe vera plant in warm weather will allow it to flourish better. Ancient Hebrew tribes used to uproot their aloe plants when they migrated, replant them upon arriving at their destination, and the plants would flourish again. With such a prestigious history, I wondered why I had not heard about Aloe Vera before. Ancient Chinese people used aloe vera gel for treating eczematous skin circumstances. It consists with a high water of nearly 96%, the aloe vera plant has been hailed as a medicinal plant with many a beneficial possessions. Ancient Chinese people used gel for treating eczematous skin circumstances. It consists of a high water content of 96% and hailed for its medicinal possessions. Studies have shown that the regular use can speed the healing process in minor wounds and serious burns. The thick leaves of the plant snap easily and can be broken off to reveal the gel inside. Studies have been conducted to observe the healing rate with various factors, such as the type of wound inflicted, it's severity and how it was bandage after applying aloe vera to it. Several of these studies have shown that the aloe vera plant does indeed speed-up the healing process overall. To get the most of aloe Vera, it's best to consume it internally to get not just external results but also internal results. When consumed as a supplement using aloeride, it helps boost your immune system and maintain your digestive tracts. This is possible because aloeride is a 100%

aloe Vera in a pill with natural ingredients that your body needs to aid it to maximum total health. Aloe Vera Product Products in their full spectrum are widely used today and gels are probably the second most frequently used product, right after Aloe vera juice. History of using it goes back probably thousands of years and it's probably one of the best known uses of nature's own force. Aloe Vera Products are known to even the skin tone and texture, diminish the appearance of pores and fine lines, and hence, make one look fresh all day.

Aloe Vera provides a deep cleaning treatment that instantly improves the problem skin by unclogging pores and removing dirt, oil and blackheads. Most aloe vera product contains pure aloe vera gel in addition to d-alpha tocopherol, triethanolamine, and methylparaben. Like Aloeride supplements when taken internally, it generally makes people feel better. This may be due to its ability to help detoxify the body. Taken daily, either alone or mixed with pure fruit juice, it is one of the best nutritional supplements available! Taken internally, Aloe Vera has been shown to have various beneficial effects on the body. It is pretty much commonplace these days. You can find in creams, shampoos, body wash, and in some cases even in toothpaste. Aloe vera gel has anti-inflammatory properties. Aloe vera contains salicylic acid that has anti-inflammatory and anti-bacterial properties. It has been used for thousands of years. It is a component of many cosmetics and burn creams. Aloe Vera is not meant to be a substitute for Western medicine but instead to act as a complement to treatment. Although I suppose even the test could turn out to be quite painful if we are. Aloe Vera, however is not just useful for its well known healing properties when applied externally, but if taken internally its benefits have been discovered to be nothing short of miraculous. The problems is that Aloe juice prepared at home from these plants is not only pretty disgusting to drink, but also cannot fully unleash the vitamins, enzymes, lignins, minerals, saponins, amino acids and anthraquinones which give the plant its potency. The gel is useful for treating athlete's foot, any forms of burns, muscular pains, herpes, eczema, pimples, bruises, diaper rash, wounds and cuts, hair loss, allergies, varicose veins, insect bites, furuncles, psoriasis, scleroderma and acne. Aloe can be used to keep the skin supple, and has also been used effectively in controlling acne and eczema. The itching which accompanies allergies and insect bites can be alleviated by using aloe

HOW TO CARE FOR ALOE VERA PLANTS

The aloe vera plant is an easy, attractive succulent that makes for a great indoor companion. Aloe vera plants are useful, too, as the juice from their leaves can be used to relieve pain from scrapes and burns when applied topically. Here's how to grow and care for aloe vera plants in your home!

Aloe vera is a succulent plant species of the genus Aloe. The plant is stemless or very short-stemmed with thick, greenish, fleshy leaves that fan out from the plant's central stem. The margin of the leaf is serrated with small teeth.

Before you buy an aloe, note that you'll need a location that offers bright, indirect sunlight (or, artificial sunlight). However, the plant doesn't appreciate sustained direct sunlight, as this tends to dry out the plant too much and turn its leaves yellow, rendering them subpar for use.

Keep the aloe vera plant in a pot near a kitchen window for periodic use but avoid having the sun's rays hit it directly.

Please note: The gel from aloe vera leaves can be used topically, but should not be ingested by people or pets. It can cause unpleasant symptoms such as nausea or indigestion and may even be toxic in larger quantities.

PLANTING

BEFORE PLANTING

• It's important to chose the right type of container. A pot made from terra-cotta or a similarly porous material is recommended, as it will allow the soil to dry thoroughly between waterings and will also be heavy enough to keep the plant from tipping over. A plastic or glazed pot may also be used, though these will hold more moisture.

• When choosing a container, be sure to pick one that has at least one drainage hole in the bottom. This is key, as the hole will allow excess water to drain out. Aloe vera plants are hardy, but a lack of proper drainage can cause rot and wilting, which is easily the most common cause of death for this plant.

• Select a container that's about as wide as it is deep. If your aloe plant has a stem, choose a container that is deep enough for you to plant the entire stem under the soil.

• Aloe vera plants are succulents, so use a well-draining potting mix, such as those made for cacti and succulents. Do not use gardening soil. A good mix should contain perlite, lava rock, chunks of bark, or all three.

• A layer of gravel, clay balls, or any other "drainage" material in the bottom of the pot is not necessary.

This only takes up space that the roots could otherwise be using. A drainage hole is drainage enough!

• (Optional) To encourage your aloe to put out new roots after planting, dust the stem of the plant with a rooting hormone powder. Rooting hormone can be found at a local garden center or hardware store, or bought online.

HOW TO PLANT (OR REPOT) AN ALOE VERA PLANT

1. Prepare your pot. After giving the new pot a quick rinse (or a good scrub, if it's a pot you've used before) and

letting it dry thoroughly, place a small piece of screen over the drainage hole; this will keep the soil from falling out the bottom and will allow water to drain properly. A doubled-up piece of paper towel or newspaper can also work in a pinch, though these will break down over time.

2. Prepare your plant. Remove the aloe vera plant from its current pot and brush away any excess dirt from the roots, being careful not to damage the roots.

If your plant has any pups, remove them now. (See the "Care" section of this page for instructions on removing and potting pups.)

If your plant has a very long, spindly stem that won't fit in the pot, it is possible to trim the stem off partially. Note that this is risky and could kill the plant. To trim the stem: Cut off part of the stem, leaving as much as possible on the plant. Next, take the bare plant and place it in a warm area that gets indirect light. After several days, a callous will form over the wound. At this point, continue with the repotting instructions below.

3. Plant your plant. Fill the pot about a third of the way with a well-draining potting mix, then place your plant in the soil. Continue filling in soil around the plant, bearing in mind that you should leave at least ¾ of an inch of space between the top of the soil and the rim of the pot. The bottom leaves of the aloe plant should rest just above the soil, too. Do not water after planting.

4. Ignore your plant (temporarily). After you've placed your aloe in its new pot, don't water it for at least a week. This will decrease the chance of inducing rot and give the plant time to put out new roots. Until the plant seems to be rooted and happy, keep it in a warm place that receives bright but indirect light.

HOW TO CARE FOR AN ALOE VERA PLANT

• Lighting: Place in bright, indirect sunlight or artificial light. A western or southern window is ideal. Aloe that are kept in low light often grow leggy.

- Temperature: Aloe vera do best in temperatures between 55 and 80°F (13 and 27°C). The temperatures of most homes and apartments are ideal. From May to September, you can bring your plant outdoors without any problems, but do bring it back inside in the evening if nights are cold.

- Fertilizing: Fertilize sparingly (no more than once a month), and only in the spring and summer with a balanced houseplant formula mixed at ½ strength.

• Repotting: Repot when root bound, following the instructions given in "Planting," above.

WATERING ALOE VERA

Watering is the most difficult part of keeping aloe vera healthy, but it's certainly not rocket science! The aloe is a succulent plant that's accustomed to arid environments, but its thick leaves still need sufficient water nonetheless.

• Water aloe vera plants deeply, but infrequently. In other words, the soil should feel moist after watering, but should be allowed to dry out to some extent before you water again. If the soil stays overly wet, the plant's roots can rot.

• To ensure that you're not overwatering your plant, allow the top third of potting soil to dry out between waterings. For example, if your plant is kept in 6 inches of potting soil, allow the top 2 inches to dry out before watering again. (Use your finger to test the dryness of the soil.)

• Generally speaking, plan to water your aloe plant about every 2-3 weeks in the spring and summer and even more sparingly during the fall and winter. One rule of thumb for fall and winter watering is to roughly double the amount of time between waterings (as compared to your summer watering schedule). In other words, if you water every two weeks in summer, water every four weeks in winter.

• When watering, some excess water may run out the bottom of the pot. Let the pot sit in this water so that the soil absorbs as much as possible. Wait 10-

15 minutes, then dump any remaining water.

REMOVING & REPLANTING ALOE VERA OFFSETS (PUPS)

Mature aloe vera plants often produce offsets—also known as plantlets, pups, or "babies"—that can be removed to produce an entirely new plant (a clone of the mother plant, technically).

1. Find where the offsets are attached to the mother plant and separate them using pruning shears, scissors, or a sharp knife. Leave at least an inch of stem on the offset.

2. Allow the offsets to sit out of soil for several days; this lets the offset form a callous over the cut, which helps to protect it from rot. Keep the offsets in a warm location with indirect light during this time.

3. Once the offsets have formed callouses, pot them in a standard succulent potting mix. The soil should be well-draining.

4. Put the newly-potted pups in a sunny location. Wait at least a week to water and keep the soil on the dry side.

HOW TO GET YOUR ALOE VERA TO FLOWER

Mature aloe vera plants occasionally produce a tall flower spike—called an inflorescence—from which dozens of tubular yellow or red blossoms appear. This certainly adds another level of interest to the already lovely aloe!

Unfortunately, a bloom is rarely achievable with aloes that are kept as houseplants, since the plant requires nearly ideal conditions to produce flowers: lots of light, sufficient water, and the right temperature range. Due to these requirements (mainly lighting), aloe flowers are usually only seen on plants grown outdoors year-round in warm climates.

To give your aloe the best shot at flowering:

• Provide it with as much light as possible, especially during spring and summer. Aloes can be kept outdoors in full sun during the summer, when temperatures are above 70°F (21°C). If nighttime temps threaten to drop below 60°F (16°C), bring the aloe inside.

Note: Don't move your aloe from indoors to full sun right away; it needs time to adjust to the intense light or it may sunburn. Allow it to sit in partial shade for about a week before moving it to a brighter location.

• Make sure the plant is getting the right amount of water—enough to keep it from drying out completely, but not enough to drown it! If the plant's being kept outdoors, make sure that it is not getting consistently soaked by summer rains.

• Give your aloe a proper dormancy period in the fall and winter. Aloe tend to bloom in late winter or early spring, so giving them a period of rest consisting of less frequent watering and cooler temperatures may encourage them to flower.

• Don't be surprised if it still doesn't flower. Despite our best efforts, indoor conditions just aren't ideal for most aloes, so don't be surprised if yours simply refuses to bloom!

PESTS/DISEASES

Aloe vera plants are most susceptible to the usual indoor plant pests, such as mealybugs and scale.

Common diseases include:

- Root rot

- Soft rot

- Fungal stem rot

- Leaf rot

Avoid overwatering to keep these conditions from developing or worsening.

HARVEST/STORAGE

ALOE VERA GEL

To make use of the aloe vera plant's soothing properties, remove a mature leaf from the plant and cut it lengthwise. Squeeze the gel out of the leaf and apply it to your burn, or simply lay the opened leaf gel-side-down on top of the affected area. Learn more about aloe vera's healing properties.

RECOMMENDED VARIETIES

Especially attractive Aloe include:

• Tiger or Partridge-Breasted Aloe (Aloe variegata) – A compact aloe characterized by short, smooth leaves with uneven white stripes.

• Lace Aloe (Aloe aristata) – A small plant with white-spotted, finely sawtoothed leaves.

• Blue Aloe (Aloe glauca) – A larger aloe species with silver-blue leaves.

Benefits of 100% Pure Aloe Vera

Aloe vera is well known plant but it is little appreciated. It has been used for medicinal and beauty purposes for centuries. It 's heeling properties are known pretty well and as early as 6500 BC it was used and acknowledged for it's curative purposes. Even then some people do not think of it as any more than a burn ointment or an analgesic gel for minor injuries, cuts and wounds. However, there are some oral 100% pure aloe vera supplements that can provide unmatched health benefits that a large proportion of people are unaware of. A better understanding of this plant comes from realizing that most of our health problems stem from a compromised digestive tract and immune system. Many people have problems in the intestinal tract and they do not even know it. When the walls of the intestines become inflamed, they let toxins and tiny food particles into the bloodstream. This is what is called the Leaky Gut Syndrome. This puts a lot of pressure on the liver and immune system since they have to constantly fight off these toxins and particles. This puts unwanted pressure on the immune system and it is compromised in the sense that when it gets occupied with fighting internal enemies it cannot resist intruders like viruses and illnesses efficiently. This is where this medicinal plant can help you considerably. It can gently clean and repair your digestive tract so that the natural balance and regularity of your intestinal and digestive properties is maintained.This is extremely crucial to your health and well being. This is because when your digestive system is working properly there is no question of it sending any toxins into the bloodstream and as a result your liver is not under undue pressure which further boosts your immune system. All this leads to well being and overall good health since the stem source of all infections is wiped off. Having mentioned the benefits of this wonder plant, it is essential for you to know that not all supplements, gels , juices etc., are of good quality. In fact there are just a few supplements that consist of 100% Pure Aloe Vera that are made

to suit the pharmaceutical standards.
Aloeride is one such supplement that
is made to suit the pharmaceutical
standards and can repair your
digestive tract to it's natural balance.
It is not only effective in treating IBS
and other digestive disorders but can
also help you get a clear and a healthy
skin. Available in pill form it is easy to
have aloe vera in the form of Aloeride
rather than in the form of juices and
gels.

Health Benefits of Aloe Vera Gel Drink

It is well known in the cosmetic and skin care industry that AloeVera has a positive effect on the skin as a healing and antiaging agent because of its ability to penetrate tissue due to its lignin content and partly due to its anaesthetic, antibacterial, antiviral, antifungal and anti-inflammatory effects. However less well known are that these effects also have a positive result on the inside of the of the body when drunk as an AloeVera Gel.

AloeVera Gel has three important qualities Nutrients and vitamins A poor diet, one that is deficient in the key elements, will not allow the body to maintain itself. Unfortunately with today's increase in fast food and ready meals most of us are likely to be short of some of items that we require. AloeVera gel is fairly unique in nature as it contains a very nutritional food, with Vitamins A, B12, C, E and Folic Acid, 19 of the 20 Amino Acids the body needs including 7 of the 8 essential amino acids and many minerals including Copper,

Manganese, Magnesium and Chromium. It also includes Lignin which aids absorption, Saponins which are soapy with antiseptic properties and Enzymes which are divided between aiding digestion and anti-inflammatory. There are also the sugars such as glucose and fructose and long-chain sugars called polysaccharides of which Acemannan is the main one. Acemannan is used in a drug to boost the immune system in animal cancer cases. Also plant sterols which are important anti-inflammatory agents and Salicylic acid which is like aspirin having pain-killing properties are contained. By drinking the gel first thing in the morning not only do you receive the benefits of the gel but also having better absorption of your breakfast. It kills bacteria, viruses, fungi and yeasts AloeVera Gel have been shown to kill or suppress certain bacteria,viruses, fungi and yeasts but its most important internally killing Candida infections in the gut. Externally it has the ability to destroy organisms that invade damaged skin and wounds, which otherwise delay or prevent healing. It is thought that probably happens internally but of course this is hard to prove. It reduces inflammation Inflammation is the normal reaction of the healthy body to injury. It involves changes to the blood supply to the wound so that molecules and cells of the immune system pass through them so the blood can clot, so starting the attack on infections and allowing the start of healing. So why do we want to reduce the inflammation? Well it is when the system goes wrong such as with hypersensitive reactions such as allergic asthma where the body over reacts and cause further damage. Or with rheumatoid arthritis, when the bodies own tissues are attacked, causing a serious degenerative condition. This is usually treated by non-steroidal anti-inflammatory drugs (NSAIDs) such as Ibuprofen, but long term use of them can have nasty side effects on the stomach such as indigestion or even bleeding stomach ulcers which can prove fatal in some cases. The properties of AloeVera gels can mean the reduction of the drugs without the stomach problems in these cases. Another very important side effect of AloeVera gel is that it helps increase the fibroblast cell replication. Fibroblast are very important in the healing process as they produce the collagen fibres of the scar tissues which knit wounds together, so the more there are the better

1.   It   contains   healthful   plant compounds

 Aloe vera may help treat skin injuries.

The cosmetic, pharmaceutical, and food industries use aloe vera extensively, and the plant has an estimated annual market value of $13 billionTrusted Source globally.

Aloe vera is known for its thick, pointed, and fleshy green leaves, which may grow to about 12–19 inches (30–50 centimeters) in length.

Each leaf contains a slimy tissue that stores water, and this makes the leaves thick. This water filled tissue is the "gel" that people associate with aloe vera products.

The gel contains most of the beneficial bioactive compounds in the plant, including vitamins, minerals, amino acids, and antioxidants.

2. It has antioxidant and antibacterial properties

Antioxidants are important for health. Aloe vera gel containsTrusted Source powerful antioxidants belonging to a large family of substances known as polyphenols.

These polyphenols, along with several other compounds in aloe vera, help inhibit the growth of certain bacteria that can cause infections in humans.

Aloe vera is known for its antibacterial, antiviral, and antiseptic properties. This is part of why it may help heal wounds and treat skin problems.

powered by Rubicon Project

3. It accelerates wound healing

People most often use aloe vera as a topical medication, rubbing it onto the skin rather than consuming it. In fact, it has a long history of use in treating sores, and particularly burns, including sunburn.

The United States Pharmacopeia describe aloe vera preparations as a skin protectant as early as 1810–1820.

Studies suggest that it is an effective topical treatment for first and second degree burns.

For example, a review of experimental studies found that aloe vera could reduce the healing time of burns by around 9 days compared with conventional medication. It also helped prevent redness, itching, and infections.

The evidence for aloe vera helping heal other types of wound is inconclusive, but the research is promising.

4. It reduces dental plaque

Tooth decay and diseases of the gum are very common health problems. One of the best ways to prevent these conditions is to reduce the buildup of plaque, or bacterial biofilms, on the teeth.

In a mouth rinse study of 300 healthy people, researchers compared 100% pure aloe vera juice with the standard mouthwash ingredient chlorhexidine.

After 4 days of use, the aloe vera mouth rinse appeared to be just as effective as chlorhexidine in reducing dental plaque.

Another study found similar benefits of aloe vera mouth rinse over a 15- to 30-day period.

Aloe vera is effective in killing the plaque-producing bacterium Streptococcus mutans in the mouth, as well as the yeast Candida albicans.

5. It helps treat canker sores

Many people experience mouth ulcers, or canker sores, at some point in their lives. These usually form underneath the lip, inside the mouth, and last for about a weekTrusted Source.

Studies have shown that aloe vera treatment can accelerate the healing of mouth ulcers.

For example, in a 7-day study of 180 people with recurrent mouth ulcers, applying an aloe vera patch to the area was effective in reducing the size of the ulcers.

However, it did not outperform the conventional ulcer treatment: corticosteroids.

In another studyTrusted Source, aloe vera gel not only accelerated the healing of mouth ulcers, it also reduced the pain associated with them.

6. It reduces constipation

Aloe vera may also help treat constipation.

This time it is the latex, not the gel, that provides the benefits. The latex is a sticky yellow residue present just under the skin of the leaf.

The key compound responsible for this effect is called aloin, or barbaloin, which has well-establishedTrusted Source laxative effects.

However, people have raised concerns about safety with frequent use. For this reason, aloe latex has not been available in the U.S. as an over-the-counter medication since 2002Trusted Source.

Contrary to popular belief, aloe vera does not appear to be effective against other digestive conditions, such as irritable bowel syndrome or inflammatory bowel disease. Learn more here.

7. It may improve skin and prevent wrinkles

There is some preliminary evidence to suggest that topical aloe vera gel can slow aging of the skin.

In a 2009 study of 30 females over the age of 45, taking oral aloe vera gel increased collagen production and improved skin elasticity over a 90-day period.

Reviews also suggest that aloe vera could help the skin retain moisture and improve skin integrity, which could benefit dry skin conditions.

8. It lowers blood sugar levels

People sometimes use aloe vera as a remedy for diabetes. This is because it may enhance insulin sensitivity and help improve blood sugar management.

For example, a review of eight studies found that aloe vera could have benefits for people with prediabetes or type 2 diabetes due to its effects on glycemic control.

However, the quality of the existing studies is not ideal, so scientists do not currently recommend using aloe vera

for this purpose

8 Uses of Alovera Gel That Would Suprise You1.

1.   Hydration

The aloe plant is very water-dense, so it's an ideal way to prevent or treat dehydration. Staying hydrated helps your body detox by providing a way for you to purge and flush out impurities. The juice also packs a hefty punch of nutrients that optimize your body's organ output.

This is crucial, because your kidneys and liver are largely responsible for the task of detoxifying your blood and producing urine. For this reason, you need to keep them healthy.

Recovery from heavy exercise also requires rehydration through the intake of extra fluids. Your body requires more fluids in order to flush and rid itself of the lactic acid buildup from exercising. Try aloe vera juice instead of coconut water after your next hard workout.

2.   Liver function

When it comes to detoxing, healthy liver function is key.

Aloe vera juice is an excellent way to keep your liver healthy. That's because the liver functions best when the body is adequately nourished and hydrated. Aloe vera juice is ideal for the liver because it's hydrating and rich in phytonutrients.

3.   For constipation

Drinking aloe vera juice helps increase the water content in your intestines. Research has shown a relationship between increasing the intestinal water content and the stimulation of peristalsis, which helps you pass stool normally.

If you're constipated or have problems with frequent constipation, try incorporating aloe vera juice into your daily routine. Aloe also helps normalize the healthy bacteria in your gut, keeping your healthy intestinal flora balanced.

4.   For clear skin

Hydrating aloe vera juice may help reduce the frequency and appearance of acne. It may also help reduce skin conditions like psoriasis and dermatitis.

Aloe vera is a rich source of antioxidants and vitamins that may help protect your skin.

The important compounds in aloe vera have also been shown to neutralize the effects of ultraviolet (UV) radiation, repair your skin from existing UV damage, and help prevent fine lines and wrinkles.

5.   Nutritious boost

Aloe vera juice is jam-packed with nutrients. Drinking it is an excellent way to make sure you don't become deficient. It contains important vitamins and minerals like vitamins B, C, E, and folic acid.

It also contains small amounts of:

- calcium

- copper

- chromium

- sodium

- selenium

- magnesium

- potassium

- manganese

- zinc

Aloe vera is one of the only plant sources of vitamin B-12, too. This is excellent news for vegetarians and vegans.

Keeping your food and drink intake nutrient-rich is key in combating most preventable diseases.

6.	Heartburn relief

Drinking aloe vera juice may give you relief when heartburn attacks. The compounds present in aloe vera juice help control secretion of acid in your stomach. The effects have even been shown to combat gastric ulcers and keep them from getting larger.

7.   Digestive benefits

Aloe vera contains several enzymes known to help in the breakdown of sugars and fats and to keep your digestion running smoothly.

If your digestive system isn't operating optimally, you won't absorb all of the nutrients from the food you're eating. You have to keep your internal engine healthy in order to reap the benefits from your diet.

Aloe vera may help decrease irritation in the stomach and intestines. The juice may also help people with irritable bowel syndrome (IBS) and other inflammatory disorders of the intestines.

One 2013 study of 33 IBS patients found that aloe vera juice helped reduce the pain and discomfort of IBS. The studyTrusted Source was not placebo-controlled, so more research is needed.

Aloe vera was also beneficial to people suffering from ulcerative colitis in an earlier double-blind, placebo-controlled study.

8.   Beauty hacks

Keeping aloe vera juice on hand can also be good for a number of beauty and health needs.

Try using it for the following:

• makeup primer (apply before foundation)

• makeup remover

• sunburn soother

• lightweight moisturizer

• treatment for irritated scalp (mix in a few drops of peppermint oil)

What are the side effects of drinking aloe vera juice?

Decolorized (purified, low anthraquinone) whole leaf aloe vera is considered safe. A 2013 study in mice fed various concentrations of purified aloe vera for three months showed no adverse effects at all from the juice.

Colored Vs. Decolorized Aloe Juice

On the other hand, nondecolorized, unpurified aloe vera juice can have unpleasant side effects, including diarrhea and cramping.

Diarrhea can lead to severe pain, dehydration, and electrolyte imbalances.

Researchers have concluded that the side effects caused by unpurified aloe vera juice are a result of the presence of anthraquinone, which is considered a laxative.

Though anthraquinone is an organic compound naturally found in the leaf of the aloe vera plant, it's considered toxic and should be avoided.

One 2013 study Trusted Source found that aloe vera whole-leaf extract increased the risk of colon adenomas (benign) and carcinomas (cancer) in rats. However, another study on rats that same year noted that purified and decolorized juice is a safer option when compared to colored aloe vera.

When shopping, look for the following statements on the label:

Purified

Decolorized

Organic

Safety tested

Drug Interactions With Aloe Vera Juice

Aloe juice has been shown to interact with certain medications. If you are taking any drug that is considered a substrate of Cytochrome P450 3A4 and CYP2D6, do not drink aloe vera juice.

Aloe vera juice may increase the risk of side effects of these drugs.

Aloe may also add to the effects of sevoflurane, causing excessive bleeding during surgery. If you are taking sevoflurane, check with your doctor before drinking aloe juice.

How Much Sugar Is In Aloe Vera Juice?

Unlike most juices, a 4-ounce serving of aloe vera juice contains no sugar and only a few calories. If you're watching your sugar intake, aloe vera juice is a healthy choice.

Amazing Uses for Aloe Vera

Aloe vera gel is widely known to relieve sunburn and help heal wounds. But did you know that your favorite potted plant can be used for much more than sunburn relief and household décor?

The succulent has a long history of being used for medicinal purposes, dating back to ancient Egypt. The plant is native to North Africa, Southern Europe, and the Canary Islands. Today, aloe vera is grown in tropical climates worldwide. From relieving heartburn to potentially slowing the spread of breast cancer, researchers are just beginning to unlock the benefits of this universal plant and its many byproducts.

Heartburn Relief

Gastroesophageal reflux disease (GERD) is a digestive disorder that often results in heartburn. A 2010 review suggested that consuming 1 to 3 ounces of aloe gel at mealtime could reduce the severity of GERD. It may also ease other digestion-related problems. The plant's low toxicity makes it a safe and gentle remedy for heartburn.

Keeping Produce Fresh

A 2014 study published online by the Cambridge University Press looked at tomato plants coated with aloe gel. The report showed evidence that the coating successfully blocked the growth of many types of harmful bacteria on the vegetables. Similar results were found in a different study with apples. This means that aloe gel could help fruits and vegetables stay fresh, and eliminate the need for dangerous chemicals that extend the shelf life of produce.

An Alternative To Mouthwash

In a 2014 study published in the Ethiopian Journal of Health Sciences, researchers found aloe vera extract to be a safe and effective alternative to chemical-based mouthwashes. The plant's natural ingredients, which include a healthy dose of vitamin C, can block plaque. It can also provide relief if you have bleeding or swollen gums.

Lowering Your Blood Sugar

Ingesting two tablespoons of aloe vera juice per day can cause blood sugar levels to fall in people with type 2 diabetes, according to a study in Phytomedicine: International Journal of Phytotherapy and Phytopharmacy. This could mean that aloe vera may have a future in diabetes treatment. These results were confirmed by another studyTrusted Source published in Phytotherapy Research that used pulp extract.

But people with diabetes, who take glucose-lowering medications, should use caution when consuming aloe vera. The juice along with diabetes medications could possibly lower your glucose count to dangerous levels.

A Natural Laxative

Aloe vera is considered a natural laxative. A handful of studies have looked into the benefits of the succulent to aid digestion. The results appear to be mixed.

A team of Nigerian scientists conducted a study on rats and found that gel made from typical aloe vera houseplants was able to relieve constipation. But another study by the National Institutes of Health looked at the consumption of aloe vera whole-leave extract. Those findings revealed tumor growth in the large intestines of laboratory rats.

In 2002, the U.S. Food and Drug Administration required that all over-the-counter aloe laxative products be removed from the U.S. market or be reformulated.

The Mayo Clinic recommends that aloe vera can be used to relieve constipation, but sparingly. They advise that a dose of 0.04 to 0.17 grams of dried juice is sufficient.

If you have Crohn's disease, colitis, or hemorrhoids you shouldn't consume aloe vera. It can cause severe abdominal cramps and diarrhea. You should stop taking aloe vera if you're taking other medications. It may decrease your body's ability to absorb the drugs.

Skin Care

You can use aloe vera to keep your skin clear and hydrated. This may be because the plant thrives in dry, unstable climates. To survive the harsh conditions, the plant's leaves store water. These water-dense leaves, combined with special plant compounds called complex carbohydrates, makes it an effective face moisturizer and pain reliever.

Potential To Fight Breast Cancer

A new study published in Evidence-Based Complementary and Alternative Medicine looked at the therapeutic properties of aloe emodin, a compound in the plant's leaves. The authors suggest that the succulent shows potential in slowing the growth of breast cancer. However, more studies are needed to further advance this theory.

Winter Proof Your Skin With Aloevera Gel

Get out the heavy woolen coats. Stoke the fireplace and take out the Aloevera gel. It's that time of year to protect yourself against the harsh elements that winter time blows our way. Taking care of our skin should be far different than when we do so during the other seasons. The cold literally zaps the moisture out of us. In turn, our skin becomes chapped and dry. Our lips are cracked and our hands burn and are blistery dehydrated You definitely are in need of winter proofing your skin and to do so with aloevera gel. There are millions of creams on the market, to be applied on the skin, that contain aloevera. Unfortunately they can only offer limited and temporary protection against the harsh weather. Working outdoors in the winter season will only prove to be unkind to your skin. In need is a powerful and potent substance that will provide skin nourishment from within and create a barrier against the cold. Cleopatra extracted the clear transparent gel from inside the leaf thousands of years ago. Today, aloevera gel has made it easier to tap into the resources only Cleopatra could dream of. The skin is made up of several layers, each with a different function. The dermis, under the top layer of the skin, is entrusted with the production of collagen which gives the skin is elasticity. Winter weather can actually hinder this production of collagen and deprive the skin's surface of the needed moisture. When deprived, the skin becomes dry and flaky. Aloevera gel triggers the production of collagen which in turn leads to healthy and young looking skin. It does this by stimulating the immune system to begin collagen production which is rich in polysaccharides. These are known to restructure the skin to keep it well protected against the harsh climate winter brings. Aloevera gel also keeps you healthy. It protects the body from hundreds of infections and diseases such as... Eczema and acne Weight loss Ulcers ...and produces a feeling of general well being. Before attempting to take care of your skin during the cold winter months, using less than perfect creams, lotions or moistures that contain less than 50% aloe vera, invest in purchasing Aloevera, a 100% natural aloevera plant condensed into a tiny pill that is easily swallowed and will provide you with countless healing properties from within. Aloe vera can be used several times a day. It works almost immediately and the results seen in a few weeks. How easy can that be? All of us strive to be as healthy as we can be and if using Aloevera will help us reach that goal, than it truly is worth the investment.

Aloe Vera For Cold and Flu

It's that time of year again when doctors all over the world advise the elderly, the vulnerable and children populations to come to their surgeries to receive an influenza vaccination (flu jab). It is very important to get this in proportion because what have these three groups in common? OK winter is here and its that period when the young and elderly are dashing into the local GP for a flue Jab. So why are these two groups vulnerable to flu?

Well the answer comes from there immune system. Their bodies immune system is either in the decline or yet to fully develop enough to fight not just flu viruses but any other kind of infection. Babies are good at sneezing at your face or socking their hands spreading the virus all over. People often mistake and confuse the difference between a flu and a cold. Cold never gives you headache or fever, you get stuffy nose, sore throat and sneezing. Sometimes chest discomfort can happen to someone with a cold. A good sign that your immune system is weak are fatigue,weakness and aches. There are claims that man often make this error than women. When you have a flue, high fever for several days is an indicator. Headache and dehydration also happens. You can experience aches, pains, fatigue and weakness. People with weak defense system can face serious effects with flu, often leading to death. History tells us that between the years 1918 and 1919 70million people was killed by flu pandemic. Its actually tragic that more people died here than did in the first world war. When you have millions of people who go about without proper nutrition due to war, the immune system can become weak, couple with the fact that sick love ones from the war also help escalate the virus. How you tackle flu depends heavily on your immune system. If you have a strong immune system, your body is able to fight the flu virus and also how quickly your system develops when under attack. People living in 1918 had weak immune system, giving in to flu viruses' that their body can't fight. So the question is, how strong is your immune system? Well most people won't know except they are put to the challenge. But how do you keep your system up and strong for defense? Here are few tips to help. First keep fit. Exercise as simple as taking a walk for up to 30mins 3 or more times a week can help. Sleep well. Go to bed early to have enough sleep. Three, eat daily nutritious food. Your body would function better when supplied with the nutrients it needs to fight the flu virus. Fresh fruits and vegetables do wonders. Grapes, vegetables, berries and aloevera supplements like aloeride are great combination. Vitamin C in 2000mg are good to improve antioxidant potential for a good defense. Viruses have a way of taking advantage of you when you're week and uprepared. Taking this steps can do a lot good. Most of them are already available by nature.

Aloe Vera Juice - The Good, Bad and the Ugly

Aloe vera juice can be used as a rub to help with muscle aches and joint pain. Applying a small amount of the juice to the area and massaging the juice into the general area of the joint is said to help the muscles relax and ease mild arthritis in the hands and elbows. It requires much more caution and should not intentionally be ingested at all. Food and Drug Administration ruled that aloe laxatives in over-the-counter drug products are not safe as it might cause problems for some people however aloe vera juice is high in antioxidants and as a result boosts a person's immune system by detoxifying the body and preventing illness. A component of aloe vera, namely acemannan, is an approved treatment for leukemia, believed to be caused by a virus similar to HIV. Aloe vera juice is also used to treat digestive problems, including heartburn, diverticular disorders and ulcers. It is antiinflammatory, which can explain why it has an effect when consumed. Medicinal uses of aloe vera are many and can improve your health considerably. It's important to note that it also prevents the causes for recurring yeast infections. It literally heals you completely. Aloe vera juices are ninety five percent water. The healing properties of aloe vera is not contained in the water of these juices, it is in the five percent of active aloe vera ingredients. Aloe vera juices made at home can alter the taste buds ability to discharge fully the anthraquinones, vitamins, lignins, enzymes, amino acids, as well as saponins that provides potency to the plant, moreover it is scabrous to consume. So it is obvious whether there is any solution or not. Aloe vera juices are used in number of lotions, creams, gels and shampoos. People can also take aloe juice as diet supplement or directly. Aloe vera juice is effective in enhancing digestive functions, restores the balance of the stomach acids. Its gel is effectively used in treating athlete's foot, any forms of burns, bruises, muscular pains, varicose veins, herpes, eczema, pimples, diaper rash, wounds and cuts, hair loss, allergies, insect bites, furuncles, scleroderma, psoriasis and acne; it also acts as antifungal. The sad truth is that aloe vera juice is one of the most adulterated health drinks on the market. Producers routinely dilute and add counterfeit chemicals, chemicals which are generally similar in molecular size to the natural elements of the juice, and which are designed to alter Standard test results. The unadulterated one's are packed full of vitamins, minerals and amino acids. All of these the body can use. While aloe vera juice has got the good and bad side of it, aloeride hasn't. No laxative or side effects. It's a better option for people who are already use to consuming aloevera juice. Though it's a pill supplement, it can also be consumed as a juice by breaking open the pill, pouring it into water. The advantage of aloeride over aloe vera juice it that fact that its not diluted with 95% water of which only the remaining 5% is aloevera . Aloeride is 100% natural aloe vera and comes with no side effects like aloe vera juice. Aloeride hasn't got any laxative effect, so it can be consumed by anyone be you allergic to laxatives or not. This is a huge advantage. Aloeride is also made to the highest quality standard, with lots of research and testing to go with it. It does all what aloe juice does and much more due to its 100% aloe content. There is nothing more added to aloeride be it additives, colouring or flavouring.

The Takeaway

There are a number of ways to use the aloe vera plant and the various gels and extracts that can be made from it. Researchers are continuing to discover new methods to put this succulent to use. Be sure to consult your doctor if you plan to use aloe vera in a medicinal manner, especially if you take medication.